Also by An...

.

The Amazing Liver & Gallbladder Flush

Timeless Secrets of Health and Rejuvenation

Cancer Is Not A Disease

Lifting the Veil of Duality

It's Time to Come Alive

Simple Steps to Total Health

Heart Disease No More

The AIDS Myth

Sunlight –The Greatest Healer of All

Sacred Santémony

Ener-Chi Art

Ener-Chi Wellness Press

Diabetes - No More!

Discover and Heal
Its True Causes

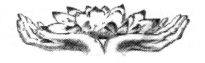

Your Health is in Your Hands

For Reasons of Legality

The author of this book, Andreas Moritz, does not advocate the use of any particular form of health care but believes that the facts, figures, and knowledge presented herein should be available to every person concerned with improving his or her state of health. Although the author has attempted to give a profound understanding of the topics discussed and to ensure accuracy and completeness of any information that originates from any other source than his own, he and the publisher assume no responsibility for errors, inaccuracies, omissions, or any inconsistency herein. Any slights of people or organizations are unintentional. This book is not intended to replace the advice and treatment of a physician who specializes in the treatment of diseases. Any use of the information set forth herein is entirely at the reader's discretion. The author and publisher are not responsible for any adverse effects or consequences resulting from the use of any of the preparations or procedures described in this book. The statements made herein are for educational and theoretical purposes only and are mainly based upon Andreas Moritz's own opinion and theories. You should always consult with a health care practitioner before taking any dietary, nutritional, herbal or homeopathic supplement, or beginning or stopping any therapy. The author is not intending to provide any medical advice, or offer a substitute thereof, and make no warranty, expressed or implied, with respect to any product, device or therapy, whatsoever. Except as otherwise noted, no statement in this book has been reviewed or approved by the United States Food & Drug Administration or the Federal Trade Commission. Readers should use their own judgment or consult a holistic medical expert or their personal physicians for specific applications to their individual problems.

ISBN: 0-9767944-6-2

Published by Ener-Chi Wellness Press – Ener-chi.com, U.S.A.
Excerpt, Timeless Secrets of Health & Rejuvenation, August 2005
Cover Design/Artwork (Ener-chi Art, Oil on Canvas, by Andreas Moritz)

Table of Contents

Understanding Diabetes – One Illness With Many Faces

At one time in recent history, many of today's epidemic disorders were well-understood to often be but symptoms of diabetes. Strokes, both ischemic and hemorrhagic, heart failure due to neuropathy as well as both ischemic and hemorrhagic coronary events, obesity, atherosclerosis, elevated blood pressure, elevated cholesterol and elevated triglycerides were all known to be common consequences of a disturbed metabolism as it occurs with diabetes. These symptoms, as well as impotence, retinopathy, renal failure, liver failure, polycystic ovary syndrome, elevated blood sugar, systemic candida, poor wound healing, peripheral neuropathy, and many others have since been turned into separate diseases, requiring specialized treatments and specialists to administer them. Although this may have greatly served the medical and pharmaceutical industry, it has led to untold suffering of patients and cost many lives unnecessarily.

Diabetes afflicts over 8% of the American population. Many of them have the belief that diabetes is inherited and the body is a victim of a genetic flaw or predisposition to the disease. Although genetic reasons can play a certain role in the manifestation of diabetes, in most cases they don't; they certainly don't explain why pancreatic cells suddenly decide to self-destruct (type I diabetes), or why common cells in people of age 50 or older for no apparent reason decide to block out insulin-laden sugar (type II diabetes).

Many patients and their doctors assume that diseases manifest because the body somehow makes a mistake and thus fails to do its job. This idea defies all sense of logic, and scientifically, it is incorrect. In this world, every effect has an underlying cause. Just because doctors are not aware of what causes pancreatic cells to stop producing insulin doesn't automatically mean this is an autoimmune disease – a disorder in which the body presumably tries to attack and destroy itself. By developing diabetes, the body is neither doing something wrong nor is it out to kill itself. It certainly finds no pleasure in making you suffer and feel miserable.

What we really should be focusing on is to create the circumstances that the body would require to shut down its insulin-producing capability in type I diabetes, and increase it in type II diabetes. With its huge number of sophisticated survival mechanisms, the body makes every effort to protect you against further harm than has already been caused through inadequate nourishment, emotional pain, and/or a detrimental lifestyle. When seen in this light, disease becomes an integral part of the body's effort to *prevent* a person from committing unintentional suicide. It can be firmly stated that your body is always on your side, never against you, even if it *appears* to attack itself (as in the so-called autoimmune disorders, such as type I diabetes, lupus, cancer and rheumatoid arthritis).

Just as there is a mechanism to become diabetic, there is also a mechanism to reverse it. To call diabetes, regardless whether it is type I or type II, an irreversible disease reflects a profound lack in understanding the true nature of the human body.

Once the preconditions for restoring balance or homeostasis have been created, the body will be able to use its full repair and healing abilities. Almost all of us know how to heal a wound or mend a broken bone. Some of us may "lose" this ability when the immune system becomes impaired, when prescription drugs interfere with blood clotting mechanisms, or when the body becomes severely congested with toxic waste matter. In the case of type I diabetes, pancreatic cells don't stop producing insulin because they are tired of doing their job. In the case of type II diabetes, the body's 60 trillion cells don't just resist the insulin that comes into contact with their cell membranes because they have developed an aversion to it. In both these situations, the cells are prevented from doing their job for a number of reasons, all of which are basically under our control. If we stop destroying the cells directly or indirectly, by the way we eat and live, they can just as easily be reprogrammed, nursed back to life or be replaced by new cells.

Healing the pancreas is not so much different than healing a broken bone. However, for healing to occur we must make certain changes that facilitate the healing, not counteract it. Treating diabetes on the symptom level prevents its cure. On the other hand, it is not difficult to determine what causes the insulin-secreting pancreatic cells to malfunction in type I diabetes, and then to remove those causes. To perform properly, these specialized cells require adequate nourishment.

Insulin is an vitally important hormone that all of us need to transport essential nutrients (proteins, sugar, fats), especially glucose, into the cells of the body. If there is not enough insulin available to deliver these nutrients to the cells, sugar, for example, becomes trapped in the blood, causing it to rise to dangerously high levels. In the case of insulin-dependent diabetes (which can occur in both types), it would seem to make sense to inject insulin into the blood in order to remove the excessive sugar, fat and protein molecules from the blood stream. However, without investigating and rectifying what has actually put the body into this awkward position, merely administering insulin shots to the patient to enforce a lower blood sugar does not only not

4

solve the problem, but, as we will see, makes it worse. This quick-fix approach actually makes a true cure impossible and, at the same time, increases the risk of developing many other ailments.

It is now known to be a fact (again) that diabetics suffering from either type have an increased risk for heart disease, cancer, stroke, blindness and Alzheimer's, etc. The question arises whether this risk is really due to the diabetes itself or its treatments. I propose that diabetes has become such a dangerous ailment because it is treated on the symptom level rather than on the causal level. If a non-insulin dependant type II diabetic receives an insulin shot, it can seriously harm or even kill him. As surprising as it may be, a healthy person who receives insulin shots will develop diabetes, which is not so uncommon, given the high percentage of false positive blood tests nowadays. "Once a diabetic, always a diabetic" is a sad consequence of medical intervention. However, it does not need to be this way.

Foods That Cause Diabetes

1. Refined Carbohydrates –
A Cause of Insulin Resistance

One of the most common guidelines given to type II diabetics is to reduce or cut out their intake of carbohydrates. They are being told that the sugars they contain may raise their blood sugar to abnormal levels and endanger their lives. While there is some truth to this statement, as we will see in the following section, it is also a dangerously misleading one. Let us first understand the true part of this statement.

It is certainly correct to say that refined, manufactured carbohydrates can seriously affect anyone's health, not just the health of diabetics. Because of the normal digestion of plant foods, the body converts complex carbohydrates into complex sugars (glycogen), which it stores in the liver and muscles. Whenever required, the body converts glycogen into glucose for generation of cellular energy. On the other hand, if you eat refined carbohydrate foods (crisps, potato chips, cakes, candy, ice cream, pasta, white bread, soft drinks, etc.), you actually bypass this process and the sugars and starches (actually, starch is sugar) they contain enter the blood stream within a matter of minutes. The more of these simple carbohydrates you consume, the higher your

6

blood sugar rises. To keep the constantly rising blood sugar in check, your pancreas has to pump extra amounts of insulin into the blood. Insulin removes sugar from the blood stream and delivers it to the cells. On the surface of the cells are insulin receptors which act as tiny doors that open and close to regulate the intake of sugar.

There is a major difference between the highly valuable glucose the body makes available to the cells and the useless sugar forced into the blood stream right after drinking a coke or eating ice cream. The cells don't like to absorb the acidic, bleached, processed and energy-stripped sugar. To protect themselves, they put up a barrier that ignores the insulin when it knocks at their door, even as it tries to deliver proper, usable quality glucose. The resulting buildup of blood sugar prompts even more insulin secretions by the pancreas, which in turn causes a larger number of cellular doors to close and blood sugar to rise further. This condition is known as "insulin resistance." When insulin production no longer keeps up with rising blood sugar, type II diabetes results. This makes type II diabetes a severe case of insulin resistance. Insulin resistance can lead to many complications in the body, including:

- Heart Disease
- Hardening of the Arteries
- Damage to Artery Walls

- Increased Cholesterol Levels
- Vitamin & Mineral Deficiencies
- Kidney Disease
- Fat Burning Mechanism Turned off
- Accumulation & Storage of Fat
- Weight Gain

2. Animal Proteins – More Harmful Than Sugar

Without a question, foods that are nutritionally empty lead to malnutrition, eating disorders and obesity. To avoid sudden, harmful blood sugar spikes, not even healthy individuals should eat refined sugar or starch-packed foods. Having a regular craving for sweets and starchy foods represents a serious signal of a major disturbance of cell metabolism. However, sugar is actually not such a big concern when you compare its effects with those caused by eating animal proteins. Diabetes patients are almost never told that the amount of insulin the body needs to process one regular piece of steak, for example, equals the amount of insulin required for about 1/2 pound of white sugar. The reason no doctor is telling you about this is that eating the steak does not substantially raise your blood sugar levels. Consequently, it appears that meat is a safe food, especially for diabetics. Because of this

8

misinformation, the "disease" can progress and worsen quietly and unnoticeably.

The insulin resistance in type II diabetics describes the condition in which the pancreas is capable of producing insulin, yet the body's cells are insensitive to it. Insulin acts as the "key" that unlocks the "gate" through which glucose and other nutrients must pass to enter cells. When there are too few "gates" open, or the "locks" on the gates are "rusted shut" and difficult to open despite the presence of insulin, insulin resistance results. Cells may actually become damaged and turn cancerous if insulin comes into contact with them too often and in excessive quantities. Regular protein meals make the cells increasingly resistant to insulin, and, without at first raising blood sugar levels, eventually lead to the high blood sugar found in type II diabetes. Frequent snacks that contain sugars and refined fats also play a major role, but as already explained, to a much lesser extent.[1] Refined fats, though, play a

---

[1] Apart from those conditions discussed here, there are other conditions which may predispose the body to the development of insulin-resistant diabetes or which may unmask a mild, subclinical, or transient diabetes that already exists. These include pregnancy, overproduction or over-administration of steroids like cortisone or prednisone, overproduction of growth hormone (acromegaly), infections, and prolonged or severe stress.

major role in type I diabetes, as we will see in section 3.

Even in a healthy body, pancreatic cells are unable to produce such large amounts of insulin as would be required for regularly consumed protein meals. Part of the unused protein is broken down by the liver, although this ability is greatly diminished in diabetics. The secreted insulin takes the rest of the protein out of the blood stream into the intercellular fluids. However, since the diabetic's cell membranes prevent insulin from entering the cells, the protein must be removed from the intercellular tissue (connective tissue) through different means. The body converts the excessive proteins into collagen fiber and stores them in the basal membranes of the blood capillary walls. This escape route leads to the common misconception that protein poses no problem for the diabetic.

Sugar, on the other hand, doesn't have such a seemingly untraceable escape route. Once the intercellular fluid is saturated with the non-absorbed sugar, it naturally rises in the blood stream. With continued protein consumption, the basal membranes accumulate so much protein fiber that simple sugars such as glucose have great difficulty passing through them. This would be the case even if the cells were to give up their insulin resistance and let the sugar pass through their membranes again. Thus, overeating protein foods makes type II diabetes a permanent blood sugar condition, a chronic illness. However, due to other food poisons the progression of this illness by no means stops here.

3. Refined Fats and Oils – Delicious Poisons?

In the 1930s, physicians considered many of our degenerative diseases to be due to a failure of our endocrine system known as *insulin resistant diabetes*. The severe derangement of the body's blood sugar control system was understood to be the basic underlying disorder that could manifest itself as nearly any kind of illness. Although there are other reasons for bringing about such a basic imbalance, as discussed before, badly engineered fats and oils are among the most influential ones. Although these fats and oils may be delicious to the taste buds, they act like poison in the body. Their destructive effects lead to severe nutritional deficiencies that prevent the body from coping with the metabolic consequences created by these poisons.

In recent years, there has been a lot of publicity about good fats and bad fats. Although some food manufacturers now claim to be able to keep bad fats out of their products, there are still thousands of common foods that contain them. The fats and oils industry still wants us to believe that the saturated fats are the bad ones, and the unsaturated fats are the good ones. This is blatantly false information. There are many highly beneficial saturated fats and just as many unhealthy unsaturated fats on the market. The only distinction that should be made when judging the value of fats is whether they are left in their natural form or are engineered. You cannot trust advertisements by the fats and oils industry that praise the amazing benefits of their unique flavorful spreads or low-cholesterol cooking fats. Their smart ad campaigns reflect zero interest in promoting your health; they are solely intended to create a market for cheap junk oils such as soy, cottonseed and rapeseed oil.

Until the early 1930s, manufactured food products were very unpopular and mostly rejected by the population because of their suspicion of them being of poor quality and not being fresh enough to be safe for consumption. The use of automated factory machinery to mass produce foods for immense potential profits was at first bitterly opposed by local farmers. Nevertheless, eventually, this resistance broke and gave way to an increasing interest in the "new" foods that no one had ever seen before. When margarine and other refined, hydrogenated products were introduced into the US food markets, the dairy industry was vehemently opposed to it, but the women found it to be more practical than the lard they had been using. Due to the shortage of dairy products during WW II, margarine became a common food among the civilian population, and the commonly used coconut oils, flax oils and fish oils disappeared from the shelves of America's grocery stores.

The campaign by the emerging food industry against natural oils and genuinely beneficial fats such as the very popular coconut oil became fueled by massive media disinformation campaigns that blamed saturated fats for the wave of heart attacks that suddenly started to grip a large portion of the American population. For 30 or more years, coconut oil was nowhere to be found in grocery stores and has only recently re-emerged in health food stores. Coconut oil and other healthful oils were practically replaced by cheap junk oils, including soy oil, cottonseed oil and rapeseed oil. While coconut fat was still the popular choice, its powerful weight-controlling effects helped prevent an obesity epidemic among the general population. Since eliminating it from the American diet, obesity has become the leading cause of illness in this country and the rest of the world.

If you are suffering from either type diabetes and wish to permanently restore your body's natural sugar-regulating mechanisms, for a certain period of time you will need to strictly avoid all artificially produced fats and oils, including those that are found in processed foods, restaurant foods, fast foods and are sold as "healthy" foods in grocery stores.

One of the most harmful oils is the genetically engineered Canola oil made from rapeseeds. Rapeseeds are not suitable for human consumption. Produced in Canada (hence the name "can-ola") this renamed, refined rapeseed oil found a huge and instant market in the U.S. during the height of the cholesterol mania (still going on). It is cheap and, therefore, widely used by restaurants and people on a low food budget. The reason for its huge popularity is that it contains very little cholesterol (which can work against the body[2]). One of the main problems with this oil is that it should not be heated; yet heating it is a standard practice in the production process, or in restaurants and households. According to a January 26, 1998 Omega Nutrition press release, "heating distorts the omega-3 essential fatty acid found in Canola, turning it into an unnatural trans form that raises total cholesterol levels and lowers HDL [good] cholesterol."

Japanese researchers found that the life spans of rats fed diets rich in Canola oil were 40% shorter. Experimental rats that were fed Canola

---

[2] Eating low cholesterol foods can dramatically increase cholesterol production in the liver. For details, see *Timeless Secrets of Health and Rejuvenation* or *Heart Disease No More!*

oil "developed fatty degeneration of the heart, kidney, adrenals, and thyroid gland." Canadian federal scientists have spent several years and a lot of money to alleviate fears linking Canola consumption to hypertension and stroke. The Health Ministry in Canada insists that although their tests match the Japanese data, Canola poses no risks to humans. Yet Canola oil consumption has been correlated with development of fibrotic lesions of the heart, lung cancer, prostate cancer, anemia, and constipation. The long-chain fatty acids found in Canola have been found to destroy the *sphingomyelin* surrounding nerve cells in the brain. Other illnesses and conditions that have been associated with Canola oil consumption include loss of vision and a wide range of neurological disorders.

How can this government be so reassuring when Canola oil has been around for a short number of years and long-term effects may not develop before 3-5 years? Is it not also strange that the FDA allowed the Canola industry to avoid the lengthy and expensive approval process, including medical research on humans? Given the alarming reactions that rats have to Canola oil, could it at least be possible that a certain percentage of heart attack and stroke victims are actually due to regular consumption of Canola oil? Since Canola oil is contained in the majority of manufactured foods, baked goods, frozen foods and restaurant foods, is it any wonder why people are falling ill everywhere, at a rate that is absolutely stunning and unprecedented?

So what do refined and manufactured oils and fats actually do to the body? For one thing, they can cause severe gastro-intestinal disturbances. The number of people in the U.S. suffering from acid reflux disease, irritable bowel syndrome, Crohn's disease, constipation, colon cancer, etc., exceeds the number of all other diseases taken together. Deep fried foods and other fast foods have become the popular choice of young people, aged 3-30. An ever-increasing number of them develop diabetes.

The high temperatures used in Canola refining and margarine production will damage many of the essential fatty acids, which are much more susceptible to damage by heat than saturated fats. Heat is known to convert many of the unsaturated double bonds to the "trans fatty acid" configuration. Although high-quality essential fatty acids as contained in some of these engineered foods are required for human health, in their damaged or rancid forms they become harmful. In fact, they may trigger power immune responses that may lead to autoimmune diseases, such as type I diabetes. The "auto-immune" part of the disease is however just a normal reaction of the immune system to the presence of these poisons that have attached themselves to cell membranes.

16

In order for cells to be healthy and functional, their plasma cell membrane, now known to be an active player in the glucose scenario, needs to contain a complement of *cis type w=3* unsaturated fatty acids. This makes the cell membranes slippery and fluid, thereby permitting glucose molecules to be able to pass through them and enter the cell interior for energy generation. This maintains balanced blood sugar levels. By regularly eating fats and oils that are heat-treated (versus natural cold pressed oils and untreated fats) the cell membranes begin to lose their healthy fatty acids and replace them with harmful trans-fatty acids and short and medium chain saturated fatty acids. As a result, the cell membranes become thicker, stiffer, sticky and inhibit the glucose transport mechanism, resulting in blood sugar rising.

The rest of the body suffers serious consequences of the clogging up of the cell membranes. The pancreas starts pumping out excessive amounts of insulin. The liver starts to convert some of the excess sugar into fat, stored by adipose cells. To get rid of the rest of the sugar, the urinary system goes into overdrive. The body goes into exhaustion due to the lack of cellular energy. The adrenals respond by pumping extra amounts of stress hormones into the blood, creating mood swings, anxiety and depression. The endocrine glands malfunction.

Overtaxed by the constant demand for extra insulin, the pancreas fails to produce enough. Body weight plummets. The heart and lungs become congested and fail to deliver vital oxygen to all the cells in the body, including the brain. Each organ and system in the body is affected by this simple dietary mistake. All this and more is what we know as diabetes, an acquired illness that can easily be avoided and even reversed by eating a natural diet consisting of natural, fresh foods that nature so generously provides for us. The idea that we can create better foods than nature does it is a fallacy that has turned into a weapon of mass destruction.

The Unfolding Drama of the Diabetes Syndrome

When sugar becomes trapped and begins to increase in the blood stream, eating sugar at this point can be life-threatening. Not having enough glucose reaching the cells and organs of the body can also be fatal. If the heart cells run out of glucose, heart failure occurs. If the kidney cells run out of glucose, kidney failure occurs. If the eyes don't get their glucose, eyesight will fail. The same applies to a sugar-starved liver, pancreas, stomach, brain, muscle, and even bone cells. By not receiving enough glucose, the body begins craving food, especially sugars, sweets, starchy foods, sweet beverages, etc., which leads to overeating and further congestion, and possibly heart congestion or cancer.

Because type II diabetes affects the health of every single one of the 60 trillion cells in the body, diabetics are predisposed to developing virtually every type of disorder there is. This has been denied by medical science for many years, but has recently been verified through major medical research. The majority of the chronic disorders plaguing our modern world today, including heart disease, cancer, arthritis, MS, Alzheimer's, Parkinson's, etc., may in actual fact not be separate diseases at all. While sharing the same cause or causes, they manifest themselves in different parts of the body as unique symptoms of disease. There will come a time when the practicing physician will recognize that diabetes, cancer, heart disease, and dementia, for example, share the same underlying causes, and therefore require the same treatment.

At the beginning stages of type II diabetes, the pancreas tries to respond to the increasing congestion of the blood vessel walls (with excessive proteins) and, possibly, to an excessive sugar or starch consumption, by secreting extra large amounts of insulin. By constantly producing disproportionate amounts of insulin, the cells become even further resistant to insulin. By blocking out insulin (along with vital nutrients) the cells try protecting themselves against the cell-damaging effects of too much insulin, or otherwise they would have to face cell mutation. Eventually, though, through intricate hormonal feedback mechanisms and enzyme signals, the pancreas recognizes both the increase in blood sugar levels and the shortage of cellular sugar, proteins and fatty acids. So the pancreas begins to deactivate, destroy or "put to sleep" a large number of its insulin-producing cells. This practically sets the stage for non-insulin dependent diabetes to become insulin-dependent diabetes.

There are a number of other reasons that may lead to reduced insulin output by the pancreas. When the basal membranes of blood capillaries supplying the pancreas with nutrients become congested with protein fiber, insulin production and other important functions, such as production of digestive enzymes, become suppressed. The same occurs when stones in the bile ducts of the liver and gallbladder drastically reduce bile secretion. In an increasing number of individuals, bile sludge consisting of small cholesterol stones enters the common bile duct and gets caught up in the *Ampulla of Vater* (where the common bile duct and pancreatic duct meet). Bile activates pancreatic enzymes before they enter the small intestine to aid in the digestion of foods. If bile flow is restricted, not all of the enzymes dispatched by the pancreas are activated. Any of these unused enzymes remaining in the pancreas can damage or destroy pancreatic cells, which leads to pancreatitis – a common cause of diabetes and pancreatic cancer. In any case, the inability of the pancreas to produce enough insulin can be a lifesaver, at least temporarily.

It is obvious, though, that this act of cancer-preventive self-preservation also means that there is not enough insulin around to transport the sugar out of the blood stream. If type II diabetics become insulin-deficient, doctors often prescribe insulin in addition to blood sugar medication, while letting them continue eating protein foods. Thus, a previously non-insulin-dependent diabetic now needs insulin shots, which greatly increases his health risks. This is completely unnecessary. I have witnessed such insulin-dependent patients turn vegan, and within just six weeks become free of the main signs and symptoms of diabetes, for the first time in 20-30 years.

Chronic disease is only chronic for as long as its causes are still intact. Insulin injection is the very thing that keeps the patient from recovering. It continues to increase the cells' resistance to insulin, and forces the pancreas to destroy an ever-increasing number of insulin-producing cells. There are plenty of natural things that can replace injection with insulin. Just one teaspoon of ground cinnamon per day can balance blood sugar. Turmeric is an amazing herb/spice with a similar effect. Broccoli and other vegetables, as well as regular full body exposure to sunlight (vitamin D-generating),[3] have superior blood sugar-regulating effects than potentially dangerous insulin injections.

Abstaining from proteins foods, cleansing the liver of stones (gallstones are a leading cause of diabetes, see details in The Amazing Liver and Gallbaldder Flush), eating a balanced diet and living a balanced lifestyle as advocated in this book are much more effective means of restoring normal body functions than just trying to fix one symptom of disease. By taking responsibility for their own health, and therefore their life, the diabetic has the opportunity to put the sweetness back into his cells and, thus, into their life.

Risks of Being Overweight

---

[3] Researchers at the University of California-Los Angeles School of Medicine (UCLA) found that compared to subjects with the highest vitamin D levels, those with the lowest levels had symptoms of type II diabetes, including weaker pancreatic function and greater insulin resistance. When the skin is exposed to ultraviolet light, the body responds by manufacturing vitamin D.

Approximately 16 million people in the United States are diagnosed with diabetes based on national statistics. In reality, through, this figure is much higher. It is estimated that another 5.4 million people have the disease and are not aware of it. Type II diabetes, also called *adult onset diabetes*, now appears routinely in six year old children. Minorities are at particular risk, as their diet consists mainly of cheap fast foods, such as hamburgers, fried chicken, pasta, potatoes, refined sweets and other highly processed foods and beverages.[4] These foods typically cause a rapid increase in blood sugar, which stimulates the production of large quantities of insulin. When there is too much insulin in the blood, the body reacts by producing the chemical *somatostatin,* which suppresses insulin release. In due time this natural response translates into diabetes.

---

[4] Researchers at the Harvard School of Public Health examined nine years of dietary and medical data on more than 51,000 women who participated in the Nurses' Health Study II. From this group, well over 700 cases of type II diabetes were diagnosed during the study period. The Harvard team concluded that the excess calories and high levels of rapidly absorbable sugars found in non-diet soft drinks promote weight gain and a greater risk of developing type II diabetes. In fact, women who drink one or more soft drinks per day may have an 80 percent increased risk of type II diabetes compared to women who avoid this type of beverage.

Compared with Caucasians, African Americans have a 60% higher risk of developing diabetes and Hispanics have a 90% increased risk. Considering the large number of undiagnosed diabetics, physicians are now losing more patients to diabetes than they are diagnosing.

An increasing number of American adults diagnosed with diabetes are obese, U.S. officials said in November 2004. A study by the Centers for Disease Control (CDC) and Prevention found that between 1999 and 2002, 54.8 percent of diabetics over the age of 19 were obese. That compared with 45.7 percent in the same age group between 1988 and 1994. When the category was expanded to include diabetics who were obese or overweight, the percentage surged to 85.2 percent in 1999-2002 compared with 78.5 percent in the earlier period. About 69 million people are obese or severely obese, according to the American Obesity Association.

In the CDC study, a person was considered overweight if their *body mass index* – the most commonly used method for calculating if a person weighs too much – was 25 to 29. Anyone with a body mass index of 30 or greater was categorized as obese. Using the body mass index to determine risk for diabetes is not completely reliable and can keep these numbers lower than they actually are. Taking averages in human statistic analysis always ends up distorting the true figures. A balanced Vata type, for example has a naturally lower weight than average. According to the body mass index Vatas are underweight. Their bones are much lighter and they have very little body fat on them. If a Vata type adds 25 pounds of body weight, it can cause him serious health problems, but according to the body mass index, this extra weight would bring him up to the normal range. Kapha types, on the other hand, have a very heavy body structure already. They cannot afford to add even 25 pounds without causing them to develop a typical Kapha disorder, such as diabetes, heart disease, or cancer.

By removing the discrepancies that exist with currently used body mass calculations, it is likely that almost every diabetic is overweight or obese. Likewise, a person who is overweight or obese can actually be considered diabetic, or at least insulin resistant. Due to the accumulation of abnormal amounts of new cells in the overweight person, there is simply not enough insulin available to meet all the nutrient demands of these extra cells. And although the pancreas may still make a normal or a little extra amount of insulin, the added weight leads to a relative insulin shortage. Eventually, the pancreas suffers from being continuously over-extended. The side-effects of a relative insulin-deficiency can be just the same as an absolute insulin-deficiency where pancreatic cells stop producing insulin altogether.

According to the American Diabetes Association, diabetes accounts for 178,000 deaths (which may not be accurate[5]), 54,000 amputees, and 12,000-24,000 cases of blindness annually. Blindness is 25 times more common among diabetic patients compared to non-diabetics. It is estimated that by the year 2010 diabetes will actually exceed both heart disease and cancer as the leading cause of death through its many complications. It is my hope that more and more scientists and doctors begin to see the strong link that exists between all these "diseases." They are metabolic disorders that share a common cause, but show up as different symptoms.

Autoimmune (Type I) Diabetes

Type I diabetes affects nearly 700,000 people in the United States. It is the most common chronic metabolic disorder to affect children. Caucasian populations, especially Scandinavians, have the greatest risk, and people

---

[5] 1 "Fast Stats" National Center for Health Statistics", Deaths/Mortality Preliminary 2001 data shows that in 2001, the most recent year for which figures US figures are posted, 934,550 Americans died from out-of-control symptoms of this disease.

26

of Asian or African descent have the lowest risk of developing this form of diabetes. Type I diabetes is usually diagnosed in children or adults under 30. The difference of risk is less due to genetic factors than to dietary ones, as we shall see shortly. Type I diabetes can develop unnoticed for years. Then, symptoms usually develop quickly, over a few days to weeks, and are caused by blood sugar levels rising above the normal range (hyperglycemia). Early symptoms include frequent urination, especially noticeable at night; possible bed-wetting among young children; extreme thirst and a dry mouth, weight loss and sometimes, excessive hunger.

Type I diabetes is defined by the absence of insulin due to the destruction of insulin-producing cells in the pancreas – called beta cells. Type I diabetics are dependent on insulin injections to control their blood sugar levels. The most common time for developing diabetes is during puberty, although it can occur at any age.

In type 2 diabetes, due to insulin resistance, the cells in the body are unable to obtain glucose that they need for energy. In type I diabetes, the cells are also deprived of glucose, but in this case, it is because insulin is not available. When cells are glucose deprived, the body breaks down fat for energy. This results in *ketones* or fatty acids entering the blood stream, causing the chemical imbalance (metabolic acidosis) called *diabetic ketoacidosis*. If left untreated, very high blood sugar would lead to flushed, hot, dry skin; labored breathing, restlessness, confusion, difficulty waking up, coma, and even death.

There is an increasing body of scientific evidence to suggest that cow's milk during childhood increases the risk of developing type I diabetes. In a recent study published in diabetes (2000), researchers found that children who had a sibling with diabetes were more than fives times as likely to develop the disorder if they drank more than half a liter (about two 8-ounce glasses) of cow's milk a day, compared with children who drank less milk.

While it is not clear which component of cow's milk may increase the risk of diabetes, researchers suspect that one of several proteins may be to blame by causing the immune system to attack insulin-producing cells in the pancreas. Dairy products so closely mimic human hormones that many times an autoimmune response is mounted. This may result in arthritis, irritable bowel, Crohn's disease, lymph edema and lymphatic congestion, phlegm in the throat, fatigue, cancer, and many other disorders.

Although many type I diabetics are known to be genetically susceptible to the disease (genetic variation), others with the same genetic variation will never develop diabetes. This suggests that dietary factors play a decisive role in who will actually become afflicted with the disorder. In fact, research showed that babies who breastfeed at least three months have a lower incidence of type I diabetes, and may be less likely to become obese as adults. This further supports and validates other research that has linked early exposure to cow's milk and cow's milk-based formula to the development of type I diabetes. Clinical studies have also shown that women who breastfeed reduce the risk of their children developing the type II diabetes.

Risky Medical Treatments

After the diagnosis of diabetes, doctors routinely prescribe either oral hypoglycemic agents or insulin. The causes of diabetes are rarely addressed, if known at all. Currently available oral hypoglycemic agents include *Biguanides, Glucosidase inhibitors, Meglitinids, Sulfonylureas* and *Thiazolidinediones*.

The biguanides lower blood sugar by inhibiting the normal release, by the liver, of its glucose stores, interfering with intestinal absorption of glucose from ingested carbohydrates, and increasing peripheral uptake of glucose. All this can completely disrupt the functions of all the organs and systems in the body.

The glucosidase inhibitors are designed to prevent the amylase enzymes produced by the pancreas to digest carbohydrates. The theory behind this is that if there is no digestion of carbohydrates the blood sugar wouldn't rise.

The meglitinides and sulfonylureas are engineered to stimulate the pancreas to produce extra insulin in a patient whose blood insulin is already elevated. Since most doctors don't measure insulin levels, this frequently prescribed drug is causing a lot of harmful side-effects, including hypoglycemia. An insulin surplus in the blood can damage blood vessels and lead to similar defects as high blood sugar.

The thiazolidinediones are known for causing liver cancer. One of them, Rezulin, was designed to stimulate the uptake of glucose from the bloodstream by the peripheral cells and to inhibit the normal secretion of glucose by the liver. After the drug killed well over 100 diabetic patients and crippled many more, it was pulled off the market.

Neither the oral hypoglycemic agents nor insulin injections have any effects on increasing the uptake of glucose by the cells of the body. This essentially means that the diabetic patient cannot expect to improve or become cured by any of these treatments. On the contrary, the prognosis with this orthodox treatment is increasing disability and early death from heart or kidney failure, or failure of some other vital organ. Research has in fact shown that diabetes drugs increase your risk of heart attack by a whooping 250%! Is it any wonder that 80% of diabetics die of heart disease?

Medical doctors don't treat you to cure your diseases. Cure is not even word they are permitted to use. Most practicing physicians and their patients want a quick fix, and in the case of type II diabetes, it consists of glucose-lowering drugs. Although these drugs can control your symptoms and lower your blood sugar, they do nothing to address the *cause* of the disorder. One of the problems with glucose-lowering drugs is that they can lose their effectiveness over time. This can dramatically increase your chances of dying from a heart attack. If that is not bad enough, these drugs can also make your life more miserable. Common side effects are weight gain, elevated cholesterol and triglyceride levels, nausea, diarrhea, constipation, stomach pain, drowsiness, and headache.

Healing the Causes

To help your body heal itself and remove the causes leading to the symptoms of diabetes (especially type II and possibly even type I), avoid eating animal proteins, such as meat, fish, poultry, eggs, cheese and cow's milk. During the recovery phase, strictly refuse consuming cheap, refined oils or fats as found in many restaurant foods and processed foods. You may use healthful fats and oils such as expeller pressed (cold pressed) coconut oil, olive oil, sesame oil and ghee butter (see your body type food list). Don't eat food that has been cooked in the microwave oven. Avoid frozen foods, canned products, and leftover foods. Take **gymnema sylvestre** to heal damaged pancreas cells, and *evening promrose oil* to improve nerve function.

Read labels. If a food contains more than 2-3 separate items on it, it is likely to be of no use for your body. Ideally, eat only foods produced by nature, such as fruits, fresh salads, cooked vegetables, grains, pulses, nuts, seeds, etc. With the exception of stevia, xylitol and D-mannose, etc., strictly avoid sugar and starchy foods such as pasta and potatoes. Much worse than sugar are artificial sweeteners and products that contain them; they should be avoided at any cost. Artificial sweeteners will reverse the recovery even if everything else is followed (see *Aspartame and Other Sweet Killer Drugs* in *Timeless Secrets of Health & Rejuvenation)*. Most vitamin supplements don't work for diabetics and may end up in the toilet. Make certain to avoid all manufactured beverages and fruit juices. Eat fruits whole, but separate from meals.

While recovering, try to monitor blood sugar manually. For some time, you may want to use glycemic tables to help you in this regard. Make sure to work with a doctor who is aware of and supportive of the healing measures you are taking for yourself. Also, avoid alcohol until blood sugar stabilizes in the normal range. The same applies to caffeine as well as other stimulants. Stimulants such as caffeine and nicotine trigger sugar release by the liver.

Those who are on the verge of developing insulin resistance or are considered pre-diabetic should follow the same guidelines. If you don't ever want to risk developing diabetes, the same guidelines apply for you also. For example, soft drinks are known to cause diabetes. Researchers at the Harvard School of Public Health examined nine years of dietary and medical data on more than 51,000 women who participated in the Nurses' Health Study II. From this group, well over 700 cases of type II diabetes were diagnosed during the study period. The study found that women who drink one or more soft drinks per day may have an 80 percent increased risk of type II diabetes compared to women who pass on this type of beverage. Changing key lifestyle factors such as diet and physical activity may not be easy for everyone. Nevertheless, in the case of controlling blood sugar, you usually have a choice. In the above study, making the choice of drinking fresh water instead of soft drinks can make the difference between life and death. If you feel you cannot make that choice, please consider that becoming diabetic can make your lifestyle much more limited and complicated than following the simple suggestions made in this book.

Diabetes is not a disease; it is a complex mechanism of protection or survival that the body takes recourse to in order to avoid the consequences of an unhealthful diet and lifestyle. Millions of people suffer or die unnecessarily from this non-disease. The diabetes epidemic is man-made, or shall I say, factory-made. It could be brought to a halt by more and more people refusing to eat foods that are not safe for human consumption.

A study, headed by Dr. Neal Barnard, compared one group of people following a low-fat vegan diet (no meat, fish, eggs, dairy, etc.) with another group on the standard American Diabetes Association (ADA) diet over 22 weeks. The results speak for themselves.

Those on the diet with no meat or dairy (compared to the ADA dieters):

- reduced their medication twice as often (43% vs. 26%)
- lost twice as much weight (14.3 vs. 7.7 lb.)
- lowered LDL-"bad" cholesterol twice as much (21.2% vs 10.7%)
- improved their Hgb A1c levels by three times as much
- cut kidney protein losses by one and a half times more

ABOUT THE AUTHOR

Andreas Moritz is a medical intuitive, a practitioner of Ayurveda, Iridology, Shiatsu and Vibrational Medicine, a writer and an artist. Born in Southwest Germany in 1954, Andreas had to deal with several severe illnesses from an early age, which compelled him to study diet, nutrition and various methods of natural healing while still a child.

By the age of 20, Andreas had completed his training in Iridology – the diagnostic science of eye interpretation – and Dietetics. In 1981, he began studying Ayurvedic Medicine in India and completed his training as a qualified practitioner of Ayurveda in New Zealand in 1991. Rather than being satisfied with merely treating the symptoms of illness, Andreas has dedicated his life's work to understanding and treating the root causes of illness. As a result of this holistic approach, he has had astounding success with cases of terminal disease where conventional methods of healing proved futile.

Since 1988, he has been practicing the Japanese healing art of Shiatsu, which has given him profound insights into the energy system of the body. In addition, he devoted eight years of active research into consciousness and its important role in the field of mind/body medicine.

Andreas Moritz is the author of *The Amazing Liver & Gallbladder Flush* (formerly, *The Amazing Liver Cleanse)*, *Timeless Secrets of Health and Rejuvenation* (formerly, *The Key to Health and Rejuvenation, Living Without Judgment* (formerly, *Freedom from Judgment) Cancer is Not a Disease* (NEW – September 2005), and *It's Time to Come Alive* (formerly, *It's Time to Wake Up)*.

During his extensive travels throughout the world, he has consulted with heads of state and members of government in Europe, Asia, and Africa, and has lectured widely on the subject of health, mind/body medicine and spirituality. His popular *Timeless Secrets of Health and Rejuvenation* workshops assist people in taking responsibility for their own health and well being. Andreas runs a free forum "Ask Andreas Moritz" on the popular health website Curezone.com (5 million readers and increasing).

After taking up residency in the United States in 1998, Andreas has been involved in developing a new innovative system of healing – *Ener-Chi Art* – which targets the very root causes of many chronic illnesses. Ener-Chi Art consists of a series of light ray-encoded oil paintings that can instantly restore vital energy flow (Chi) in the organs and systems of the body. Andreas is also the founder of Sacred *Santèmony – Divine Chanting for Every Occasion,* a powerful system of specially generated frequencies of sound that can transform deep-seated fears, allergies, traumas and mental/emotional blocks into useful opportunities of growth and inspiration within a matter of moments.

Other Books, Products and Services By The Author

Timeless Secrets of
Health and Rejuvenation –
Breakthrough Medicine for the 21st
Century (500 pages)

This book meets the increasing demand for a clear and comprehensive guide that can help make people self-sufficient regarding their health and well-being. It answers some of the most pressing questions of our time: How does illness arise? Who heals, who doesn't? Are we destined to be sick? What causes aging? Is it reversible? What are the major causes of disease and how can we eliminate them?

Topics include: The placebo and the mind/body mystery; the laws of illness and health; the four most common risk factors of disease; digestive disorders and their effects on the rest of the body; wonders of our biological rhythms and how to restore them if disrupted; how to create a life of balance; why to choose a vegetarian diet; cleansing the liver, gallbladder, kidneys and colon; removing allergies; giving up smoking naturally; Using sunlight as medicine;

the 'new' causes of heart disease, cancer and AIDS; and antibiotics, blood transfusions, ultrasounds scans, immunization programs under scrutiny.

Timeless Secrets of Health and Rejuvenation sheds light on all the major issues of health care and reveals that most medical treatments, including surgery, blood transfusions, pharmaceutical drugs, etc., are avoidable when certain key functions in the body are restored through the natural methods described in the book. The reader also learns about the potential dangers of medical diagnosis and treatment as well as the reasons vitamin supplements, 'health' foods, light products, 'wholesome' breakfast cereals, diet foods and diet programs may have contributed to the current health crisis rather than helped resolve it. The book includes a complete program of health care, which is primarily based on the ancient medical system of Ayurveda and the vast amount of experience Andreas Moritz has gained in the field of health during the past 30 years.

The Amazing Liver & Gallbladder Flush
A Powerful Do It Yourself Tool to Optimize your Health and Wellbeing

In this revised edition of his best selling book, *The Amazing Liver Cleanse,* Andreas Moritz addresses the most common but rarely recognized cause of illness – gallstones congesting the liver. Twenty million Americans suffer from attacks of gallstones every year. In many cases, treatment merely consists of removing the gallbladder, at the cost of $5 billion a year. However, this purely symptom-oriented approach does not eliminate the cause of the illness, and in many cases, sets the stage for even more serious conditions. Most adults living in the industrialized world, and especially those suffering a chronic illness such as heart disease, arthritis, MS, cancer, or diabetes, have hundreds if not thousands of gallstones (mainly clumps of hardened bile) blocking the bile ducts of their liver.

This book provides a thorough understanding of what causes gallstones in the liver and gallbladder and why these stones can be held responsible for the most common diseases so prevalent in the world today. It provides the reader with the knowledge needed to recognize the stones and gives the necessary, do-it-yourself instructions to painlessly remove them in the comfort of one's home. It also gives practical guidelines on how to prevent new gallstones from being formed. The widespread success of *The Amazing Liver & Gallbladder Flush* is a testimony to the power and effectiveness of the cleanse itself. The liver cleanse has led to extraordinary improvements in health and wellness among thousands of people who have already given themselves the precious gift of a strong, clean, revitalized liver.

Lifting the Veil of Duality –
Your Guide to Living without Judgment

"Do you know that there is a place inside you -- hidden beneath the appearance of thoughts, feelings and emotions – that does not know the difference between good and evil, right and wrong, light and dark? From that place, you embrace the opposite values of life as *One*. In this sacred place you are at peace with yourself and at peace with your world." *Andreas Moritz*

In *Lifting the Veil of Duality*, Andreas Moritz poignantly exposes the illusion of duality. He outlines a simple way to remove every limitation that you have imposed upon yourself during the course of living duality. You will be prompted to see yourself and the world through a new lens – the lens of clarity, discernment and non-judgment. And you will find out that mistakes, accidents, coincidences, negativity, deception, injustice, wars, crime and terrorism all have a deeper purpose and meaning in the larger scheme of things. So naturally, much of what you will read may conflict with the beliefs you currently hold. Yet you are not asked to change your beliefs or opinions. Instead, you are asked to have *an open mind,* for only an open mind can enjoy freedom from judgment.

Our personal views and worldviews are currently challenged by a crisis of identity. Some are being shattered altogether. The collapse of our current World Order forces humanity to deal with the most basic issues of existence. You can no longer avoid taking responsibility for the things that happen to you. When you *do* accept responsibility, you also empower and heal yourself.

Lifting the Veil of Duality shows you how you create or subdue your ability to fulfill your desires. Furthermore, you will find intriguing explanations about the mystery of time, the truth and illusion of reincarnation, the misleading value of prayer, what makes relationships work and why so often they don't. Find out why injustice is an illusion that has managed to haunt us throughout the ages. Learn about our original separation from the Source of life and what this means with regard to the current waves of instability and fear so many of us are experiencing.

Discover how to identify the angels living amongst us and why we all have light-bodies. You will have the opportunity to find the ultimate God within you and discover why a God seen as separate from yourself keeps you from being in your Divine Power and happiness. In addition, you can find out how to heal yourself at a moment's notice. Read all about the "New Medicine" and the destiny of the old medicine, the old economy, the old religion and the old world.

It's Time to Come Alive!
Start Using the Amazing Healing Powers of Your Body, Mind and Spirit Today!

In this book, the author brings to light man's deep inner need for spiritual wisdom in life and helps the reader develop a new sense of reality that is based on love, power and compassion. He describes our relationship with the natural world in detail and discusses how we can harness its tremendous powers for our personal and humankind's benefit. *Time to Come Alive* challenges some of our most commonly held beliefs and offers a way out of the emotional restrictions and physical limitations we have created in our lives.

Topics include: What shapes our Destiny; using the power of intention; secrets of defying the aging process; doubting - the cause of failure; opening the heart; material wealth and spiritual wealth; fatigue – the major cause of stress; methods of emotional transformation; techniques of primordial healing; how to increase health of the five senses; developing spiritual wisdom; the major causes of today's earth changes; entry into the new world; twelve gateways to heaven on earth; and many more.

Cancer is Not a Disease!
Discover the Hidden Purpose of Cancer, Heal its Underlying Causes, and Let Your Body Take Care of the Rest

This latest book by Andreas Moritz may rock or even dismantle the very foundation of your beliefs about the body, health and healing. It offers the open-minded reader concerned about cancer a radically different understanding of what cancer really is. According to Andreas Moritz, cancer is a desperate and final attempt by the body to stay alive for as long as circumstances permit – circumstances that are, in fact, in your control.

Today's conventional approaches of killing, cutting or burning cancerous cells offer a mere

7% "success" rate for cancer remission, and the majority of the few survivors are "cured" for just a period of five years or less. In this book, you will discover what actually causes cancer and why it is so important to heal the whole person, not just the symptom of cancer. You will also learn that cancer occurs only after all other defense mechanisms in the body have failed, for obvious reasons. A malignant tumor is not a vicious monster that is out to kill us in retaliation for our sins or abuse of our body. As you will find out, cancer is not attempting to kill the body; to the contrary, the cancer is trying to save it. However, unless we change our perception of what cancer really is, it will continue threatening the life of one out of every two people. This book opens a door to those who wish to become complete again, in body, mind and spirit.

Topics of the book include:
- Reasons that coerce the body to develop cancer cells
- How to identify and remove the causes of cancer
- Why most cancers disappear by themselves, without medical intervention
- Why radiation, chemotherapy and surgery never cure cancer

- Why some people survive cancer *despite* undergoing dangerously radical treatments
- The roles of fear, frustration, low self-worth and repressed anger in the origination of cancer
- How to turn self-destructive emotions into energies that promote health and vitality
- Spiritual lessons behind cancer

Simple Steps to Total Health!
With co-author John Hornecker

By nature, your physical body is designed to be healthy and vital throughout life. Unhealthy eating habits and lifestyle choices, however, lead to numerous health conditions that prevent you from enjoying life to the fullest. In *Simple Steps to Total Health*, the authors bring to light the most common cause of disease, which is the build-up of toxins and residues from improperly digested foods that inhibit various organs and systems from performing their normal functions. This guidebook for total health provides you with simple but highly effective approaches for internal cleansing, hydration, nutrition and living habits.

The book's three parts cover the essentials of total health – Good Internal Hygiene, Healthy Nutrition and Balanced Lifestyle. Learn about the most common disease-causing foods, dietary habits and influences responsible for the occurrence of chronic illnesses, including those affecting the blood vessels, heart, liver, intestinal organs, lungs, kidneys, joints, bones, nervous system and sense organs.

To be able to live a healthy life, you must align your internal biological rhythms with the larger rhythms of nature. Find out more about this and many other important topics in *Simple Steps to Total Health*. This is a "must-have" book for anyone who is interested in using a natural, drug-free approach to restoring total health.

Heart Disease No More!
Make Peace with Your Heart and Heal Yourself

Less than one hundred years ago, heart disease was an extremely rare disease. Today it kills more people in the developed world than all other causes of death combined. Despite the vast amount of financial resources spent on finding a cure for heart disease, the current medical approaches remain mainly symptom-oriented and do not address the underlying causes.

Even worse: There is overwhelming evidence to show that the treatment of heart disease or its presumed precursors, such as high blood pressure, hardening of the arteries and high cholesterol, does not only prevent a real cure but can easily lead to chronic heart failure. The patient's heart may still beat, but not strong enough to feel vital and alive.

Without removing the underlying causes of heart disease and its precursors, there is little, if any, protection against it. Heart attacks can strike regardless whether you have had a coronary bypass done or stents placed inside your arteries. According to research, these procedures fail to prevent heart attacks or reduce mortality rates.

Heart Disease No More, excerpted from the author's bestselling Timeless Secrets of Health & Rejuvenation, puts the responsibility for healing where it belongs, that is, to the heart, mind and body of each individual. It provides you with the practical insights about how heart disease develops, what causes it and what you can do to prevent and reverse it for good, regardless of a possible genetic predisposition.

**All books are available as paperback copies
and electronic books
through the Ener-Chi Wellness Center.
Website: http://www.ener-chi.com
Email: andmor@ener-chi.com
Phone: (615) 676-9961 or (864) 848 6410**

Sacred Santémony – for Emotional Healing

Sacred Santémony is a unique healing system that uses sounds from specific words to balance deep emotional/spiritual imbalances. The powerful words produced in Sacred Santémony are made from whole-brain use of the letters of the *ancient language* – language that is comprised of the basic sounds that underlie and bring forth all physical manifestation. The letters of the ancient language vibrate at a much higher level than our modern languages, and when combined to form whole words, they generate feelings of peace and harmony (Santémony) to calm the storms of unrest, violence and turmoil, both internal and external.

In April 2002, I spontaneously started chanting sounds that are meant to improve certain health conditions. These sounds resembled chants by Native Americans, Tibetan monks, Vedic pundits (Sanskrit) and languages from other star systems (not known on planet Earth). Within two weeks, I was able to bring forth sounds that would instantly remove emotional blocks and resistance or aversion to certain situations and people, foods, chemicals, thought forms, beliefs, etc. The following are but a few examples of what Sacred Santémony may be able to assist you with:

- Reducing or removing fear that is related to death, disease, the body, foods, harmful chemicals, parents and other people, lack of abundance, impoverishment, phobias, environmental threats, the future and the past, unstable economic trends, political unrest, etc.
- Clearing or reducing a recent or current hurt, disappointment or anger resulting from past emotional trauma or negative experiences in life.
- Cleansing of the *Akashic Records* (a recording of all experiences the soul has gathered throughout all life streams) from persistent fearful elements, including the idea and concept that we are separate from and not one with Spirit, God or our Higher Self.
- Setting the preconditions for you to resolve your karmic issues not through pain and suffering, but through creativity and joy.
- Improving or clearing up allergies and intolerances to foods, chemical substances, pesticides, herbicides, air pollutants, radiation, medical drugs, pharmaceutical byproducts, etc.
- Undoing the psycho-emotional root causes chronic illnesses, including

cancer, heart disease, MS, diabetes, arthritis, brain disorders, depression, etc.

- Resolving other difficulties or barriers in life by "transforming" them into the useful blessings that they really are.

To arrange for a personal Sacred Santémony session with Andreas Moritz, please follow the same directions as given for Telephone Consultations.
(See fees under "Telephone Consultations)

Ener-Chi Art

In collaboration with Dr. Lillian Maresch, Andreas Moritz has developed a new system of healing and rejuvenation designed to restore the basic life energy (Chi) of an organ or a system in the body within a matter of seconds. Simultaneously, it also helps balance the emotional causes of illness.

Eastern approaches to healing, such as Acupuncture and Shiatsu, are intended to enhance well-being by stimulating and balancing the flow of Chi to the various organs and systems of the body. In a similar manner, the energetics of Ener-Chi Art is designed to restore a balanced flow of Chi throughout the body.

According to most ancient systems of health and healing, the balanced flow of Chi is the key determinant for a healthy body and mind. When Chi flows through the body unhindered, health and vitality are maintained. By contrast, if the flow of Chi is disrupted or reduced, health and vitality tend to decline.

A person can determine the degree to which the flow of Chi is balanced in the body's organs and systems by using a simple muscle testing procedure. To reveal the effectiveness of Ener-Chi Art, it is important to apply this test both before and after viewing each Ener-Chi Art picture.

To allow for easy application of this system, Andreas has created a number of healing paintings that have been "activated" through a unique procedure that imbues each work of art with specific color rays (derived from higher the higher dimensions). To receive the full benefit of an Ener-Chi Art picture all that is necessary is to look at it for less than a minute. During this time, the flow of Chi within the organ or system becomes fully restored. When applied to all the organs and systems of the body, Ener-Chi Art sets the precondition for the whole body to heal and rejuvenate itself.

Ener-Chi Ionized Stones

Ener-Chi Ionized Stones are stones and crystals that have been energized, activated, and imbued with life force through a special process introduced by Dr. Lillian Maresch and Andreas Moritz -- the founders of Ener-Chi Art.

Stone ionization has not been attempted before because stones and rocks have rarely been considered useful in the field of healing. Yet, stones have the inherent power to hold and release vast amounts of information and energy. And, once ionized, they exert a balancing influence on everything with which they come into contact. The ionization of stones may be one of our keys to survival in a world that is experiencing high-level pollution and destruction of its eco-balancing systems.

In the early evolutionary stages of Earth, every particle of matter within the mantle of the planet contained within it the blueprint of the entire planet, just as every cell of our body contains within its DNA structure the blueprint of our entire body. The blueprint information within every particle of matter is still there – it has simply fallen into a dormant state. The ionization process "reawakens" this original blueprint information, and enables the associated energies to be released. In this sense, Ener-Chi Ionized Stones are alive and conscious, and are able to energize, purify and balance any natural substance with which they come into contact.

By placing an Ionized Stone next to a glass of water or plate of food, the water or food becomes energized, increasing digestibility and nutrient absorption. Ionized stones can also be used effectively in conjunction with Ener-Chi Art – simply place an Ionized Stone on the corresponding area of the body while viewing an Ener-Chi Art picture.

Potential Uses for Ionized Stones

Drinking Ionized Water
Placing an Ionized Stone next to a glass of water for about half a minute ionizes the water. Ionized water is a powerful cleanser that aids digestion and metabolism, and energizes the entire body.

Eating Ionized Foods
Placing an Ionized Stone next to your food for about half a minute ionizes and balances it. Even natural organic foods are usually somewhat polluted due to the pollution particles in our atmosphere and soil. Such foods also are impacted by ozone depletion and exposure to electro-magnetic radiation in our planetary environment. These negative effects tend to be

neutralized through the specified use of Ionized Stones.

Ionized Foot Bath

By placing Ionized Stones (preferably pebbles with rounded surfaces) under the soles of the feet, while the feet are immersed in water, the body begins to break down toxins and waste materials into harmless organic substances.

Enhancing Healing Therapies

Ionized Stones are ideal for enhancing the effects of any healing therapy. For example, "LaStone Therapy" is a popular new therapy that is offered in some of the innovative health spas. This involves placing warm stones on key energy points of the body, as shown in the picture. If these stones were ionized prior to being placed on the body, the healing effects would be enhanced. In fact, placing Ionized Stones on any weak or painful part of the body, including the corresponding chakra, has healthful benefits. If crystals play a role in the therapy, ionizing them first greatly amplifies their positive effects.

Aura and Chakra Balancing

Holding an Ionized Stone or Ionized Crystal in the middle section of the spinal column for about one-half minute balances all of the chakras, or energy centers, and tends to keep them in balance for several weeks, or even months. Since energy imbalances in the chakras and auric field are one of the major causes of health problems, this balancing procedure is a powerful way to enhance health and well-being.

Attach to Main Water Pipe in Your Home

Attaching a stone to the main water pipe will ionize your water and make it more absorbable and energized.

Place In, or Near, Electrical Fuse Box in Your Home

By placing a larger Ionized Stone in, above or below the fuse box in your house, the harmful effects of electromagnetic radiation become nullified. You can verify this by doing the muscle test (as shown in the instruction sheet of Ener-Chi Art) in front of a TV or computer, both before and after placing the stone on the fuse box. If you don't have a fuse box that is readily accessible, you can place a stone next to the electric cable of the electric appliances or the power sockets.

Use in Conjunction with Ener-Chi Art

Ionized Stones may be used to enhance the effects of Ener-Chi Art pictures. Simply place an Ionized Stone over the related area of the body while viewing an Ener-Chi Art picture. For example, if one is viewing the Ener-Chi Art picture related to the heart, simply hold an ionized stone over the heart area while viewing the picture. The nature of the energies involved in the pictures and the stones is similar. So if the stones are used in combination with the pictures, a resonance is created which greatly enhances the overall effect.

Creating an Enhanced Environment

Placing an Ionized Stone near the various items that surround you for about half a minute helps to create a more energized and balanced environment. The Ionized Stones affect virtually all natural materials, such as wood floors, wood or metal furniture, stone walls, and brick or stone fireplaces. In work areas, especially near computers, it is a good idea to place one or more Ionized Stones in strategic locations. The same applies to sleeping areas, such as putting stones under your bed or pillow.

Improving Plant Growth

Placing Ionized Stones next to a plant or flower pot may increase their health and beauty. This automatically ionizes the water they receive, whether they are indoor or outdoor plants. The same applies to vegetable plants and organic gardens.

Creating More Ionized Stones

Make any number of ionized stones simply by holding your "seed stone" against any other stones or crystals for 40-50 seconds. Your new stones will have the same effect as the seed stone.

Telephone Consultations

For a Personal Telephone Consultation with Andreas Moritz, please

1. Call or send an email with your name, phone number, address (digital picture of your face if you have one) and any other relevant information to Andreas.

2. Set up an appointment for the length of time you choose to spend with him. A comprehensive consultation lasts 2 hours or more. Shorter consultations deal with all the questions you may have and the information that is relevant to your specific health issue(s).

Fees (September 2006**):** $110 for 1/2 hour, $225 for one hour, $335 for 1 1/2 hours, and $445 for 2 hours (fees are subject to change).

Note: Shorter consultations deal with all the questions you may have and the information that is relevant to your specific health issue(s). For a comprehensive consultation, (if you have a digital camera) please take a snapshot of your face (preferably without makeup) and email it to Andreas before your appointment with him. This can greatly assist Andreas in assisting you in your quest for better health.

To order Ener-chi Art pictures, Ionized Stones, and other products

please contact:

Ener-Chi Wellness Center, LLC

Web Site: http://www.ener-chi.com
E-mail: enerchiart@aol.com

Phone: (864) 848-6410 (USA)
EVoice: (615) 676-9961 (USA)